Also by Dr. Stenbeck

Available from the usual on-line source

The Pallinomic Body Type

The President Johnson, Jane Russell Celebrity Body Type

For Kaye,
there at the beginning with Doc Severn,
and for Liberty,
continuing the holistic healing journey…

About the Author

Educated in New Zealand and in the U.S.A., Dr. Stenbeck attained B.Sc. (NZ), M.S., and D.C. degrees. His holistic healing methods have been profiled in magazines (Esquire, McLean's, Playgirl, the Atlanta Constitution), and on TV in the USA and in Canada. He was the main contributor to the Warner Book, _The Eye/Body Connection_ by Jessica Maxwell that focused on the holistic healing relationships between the iris structure and organ genetics.

In the 1970-80's he was elected Fellow, Royal Society of Health, London; Fellow, American Association of Chemists; Member, American Association of Clinical Chemists; and Affiliate, Royal Society of Medicine, London. He studied naturopathy and Body Types with Dr. Bernard Jensen and Dr. Clifford Severn, and has practiced in medical partnerships where patients received the joint benefits of medical and holistic healing.

He is a member of Self-Realization Fellowship. To receive advice on any health issue from a holistic viewpoint, or to receive help with your body type, see his web site: *DrStenbeck.net*

———

Contents

* * *

The Pallinomic Body Type and Food Guide   1

<u>*Appendix*</u>

* * *

The 22 Body Types:
Celebrity Examples

This Booklet contains the **Pallinomic** *type.
See* <u>The 22 Unique Body Types</u> *for all type
descriptions.]*

———

Thin Types

Atrophic   *Woody Allen / Audrey Hepburn
Stan Laurel / Calista Flockheart*

Exesthesic   *Cher / Sarah Jessica Parker
(Female type only)*

Marasmic   *President Obama / Princess Diana
James Stewart / Kate Blanchard*

Neurogenic   *J.K. Simmons / Joan Rivers
Jon Cryer / Marin Hinle*

Pathoferic   *(No celebrity males)
Blythe Danner / Gwyneth Paltrow*

Sillevitic   *David Bowie / Shirley MacLaine
Rod Stewart / Carol Channing*

Muscle Types

Calciferic   *Michael Jordan / Angelica Huston*
          Abraham Lincoln / Grace Jones

Carbogenic   *George Clooney / Lady Gaga*
          Pres. Trump / Meg Ryan

Desmogenic   *Marlon Brando / Loni Anderson*
          Daniel Craig / Tina Turner

Eldic   *Ross Perot / Hillary Clinton*
          Peter Falk / Sigourney Weaver

Myogenic   *Pres. Bill Clinton / Sharon Stone*
          Pres. John Kennedy / Julia Roberts

Nervimotive *Frank Sinatra / Elizabeth Taylor*
          Mark Wahlberg / Natalie Wood

Nitropheric *Ben Affleck / Ava Gardner*
          Kirk Douglas / Kate Winslet

Pallinomic   *Pres. Lyndon Johnson /*
          Attorney General Janet Reno
          Bill O'Reilly (Fox) / Jane Russell

Muscle Types

Calciferic	*Michael Jordan / Angelica Huston Abraham Lincoln / Grace Jones*
Carbogenic	*George Clooney / Lady Gaga Pres. G. Bush, Jr. / Meg Ryan*
Desmogenic	*Marlon Brando / Loni Anderson Daniel Craig / Tina Turner*
Eldic	*Ross Perot / Hillary Clinton Peter Falk / Sigourney Weaver*
Myogenic	*Pres. Bill Clinton / Sharon Stone Pres. John Kennedy / Julia Roberts*
Nervimotive	*Frank Sinatra / Elizabeth Taylor Mark Wahlberg / Natalie Wood*
Nitropheric	*Ben Affleck / Ava Gardner Kirk Douglas / Kate Winslet*
Pallinomic	*Pres. Donald Trump / Attorney General Janet Reno Bill O'Reilly (Fox) / Jane Russell*

Fat Types

Barotic *Robin Williams / 'Mrs.Doubtfire'*
Elton John / William Conrad

Carboferic *Bill Murray / Roseanne*
Billy Gardell / Melissa McCarthy

Hydripheric *John Goodman / Shelly Winters*
Wayne Knight / Jennifer Holliday

Isogenic *Einstein / Oprah Winfrey*
Phillip S .Hoffman / Queen Victoria

Lipopheric *Rush Limbaugh / Rosie O'Donnell*
Chris Christie / Camryn Manheim

Oxypheric *Winston Churchill / Orsen Welles*
Ella Fitzgerald / Gerry Spence

Pargenic *Burt Reynolds / Katey Segal*
Ron Perlman / Kirstey Alley

Succinct Quote on Human Types

From Victor Rocine, who first described discrete body types around 1900.

"A type is an order of people that differentiates and distinguishes itself by a general and similar form, brain-formation, chemistry, structure, build, immunity, tendencies, predisposition, resemblance, skin-pigment, and type characteristics based on observation and analogy.

"Or, in other words, people of a given type are similar physically and like-minded as if they were brothers and sisters—that is what type means.

"Everything in nature is made according to plan. Man only discovers that plan and gives it a name. The zoologist has not made the animals—he has only described the plan adopted by the wonderful Creator, and named the classes, sub-classes, etc.

"How important type research will be to humanity, time alone will make known."

———

Prologue

The esteemed scientist J. J. Berzelius, discoverer of several chemical elements, inspired Victor Rocine to research body types and to investigate the correlation between types and their diseases. Around 1890-1910, Rocine privately published his original findings on the mineral basis of different body types, and this present book exists because of his brilliant insights.

For many years, I studied with Dr. Clifford Severn who had been a personal student of Victor Rocine on body types, naturopathy, herbology, iris analysis, diet, and nutritional healing methods. He had a successful career as a lecturer and healer, and was one of those rare athletes with complete muscle control over his body. I saw him under a spotlight at 85 years of age, contracting and rippling every individual muscle in his perfectly developed body. Field-Marshal Jan Smuts, the WWII South African Prime Minister, devoted a full chapter of his autobiography to how Severn's healing methods had saved his life. In the 1950's, *Life* magazine did a four-page spread on Severn and his family. Fame he had.

Another Rocine student I studied with, Dr. Bernard Jensen wrote of Rocine's body type research and nutritional methods in his privately published book *The Chemistry of Man*.

This book is deeply rooted in Rocine's original work, and with that of Herbert Shelton, M.D., Ph.D. (at Harvard University in the 1930's). I integrated their research with newer dietary and nervous system data along with celebrity examples of each type, hopefully, making this material easier to digest and more entertaining for the reader.

Gayelord Hauser, another Rocine student I knew, was a celebrated health book author. He wrote a popular book on Rocine's types in the 1940's, *Types and Temperaments;* reputedly, he also introduced yogurt to the western world.

This book exists because of Rocine's creative brilliance and original discoveries in natural healing.

▶ *Rocine: "The soul creates the body type."*

Rocine taught that the soul chooses a body type and brain to live in, thus presenting different experiences and life lessons to master. Why were *you* born the way you are?

That is something to think about, especially if it is true! What would your soul purpose be to live in a particular body type. I provide some thoughts on this issue in each type description and try to assess from my experience with your type the particular lessons of life presented therein.

Rocine was as brilliant in his way as an Abraham Lincoln, Michael Jordan, Michael Phelps, or Tony Robbins—all *calciferic* types—rare, leaders, innovative, brilliant, and highly intelligent in their different fields of endeavor.

Celebrity examples exist for most types, not a duplicate of you, but someone who has your essence in their body-mind individuality. Knowing your type allows you to become a better you!

The celebrity examples provide further help in identifying your body type.

▶ *Rocine's classic findings are the backbone of this book. Integrated with Sheldon's research and with other dietary and food issues including mental, emotional, and spiritual attributes,*

Many people take nutritional supplements and try different diets without a doctor's advice. If this is your choice, use common sense, listen to body responses, and discontinue any allergic reactions to foods or nutritional substances.

———

The Pallinomic Body Type

Representing one of the 22 Body Types first described by Victor Rocine around 1900

* * *

"You may also have a physical or psychological feature not representative of your type such as height, weight, appearance, talent, weakness, strength, etc., due to biochemical errors, environmental influences, racial or cultural differences, and congenital or genetic issues. Nevertheless, the type identification of the average person is usually clear."

— *Victor Rocine*

Pallinomic Type Celebrity Examples

*If you think this is your type, be sure to look at **on-line photographs** of these examples. Look for general similarities to yourself. Note that sub-types cause the differences in appearance between members of the same type.*

GOVERNMENT

President Theodore Roosevelt
President Lyndon Johnson
President Ronald Reagan
Attorney General Janet Reno
[Note – The pallmomic type is President Trump's subtype.]

ACTORS/TV

Bill O'Reilly (Fox)
Buddy Epsen
Rock Hudson
Victor Mature
Lorne Greene
Claude Aitkins
Craig T. Nelson
Clint Walker
Broderick Crawford

Liam Nielsen
John Wayne
Randy Quaid
Robert Mitchum
Johnny Weismuller
Ken Howard
Andy Griffin
Ward Bond
Fes Parker

James Gandolfino   Gerard Depardieu
James Arness   Ed McMann
Ed O'Neil   Paul Drake
Camryn Manheim   Jane Russell
Rosemary Clooney
Brenda Blethyn (BBC's "Vera")

SPORTS

Ted Williams   Greg Norman
Don Drysdale (Dodgers) Don Shula
Lindsay Davenport (Tennis)

ARTS/OTHER

Dave Brubeck   Adelle
Susan Boyle   Julia Childs
Ina Garten (TV Cooking) Fabio

[Note: I personally knew numerous members of this type in everyday life, and a family member, which contributed to my understanding of the type.]

Read the types, and if still confused you may choose to use the personal request for type identification from my web site: *DrStenbeck.net*

▶ *My celebrity type identifications, mostly from photos and movies,* **cannot** *be 100% accurate, and I assess my typing at about 80% accurate.*

———

Pallinomic Type Questionnaire

Other than for the physical descriptions, these questions describe the generic type, and not specifically you! If any question ever applied to you, then choose he True answer!

For Question 1 only:

A = True	*B = Maybe*	*C = Untrue*
15 points	*7 points*	*1 point*

1. Physically identify with celebrity example _____

Then...

A = True	*B = Maybe*	*C = Untrue*
5 points	*3 points*	*1 point*

---

2. Height is close to:
   Males: 5'10-6'8   Females: 5'7-6'2   _____
3. Usual weight is close to:
   Males: 170-300+   Females: 160-300+   _____
4. Body medium-sized when young;
   then invariably heavy; pot-bellied males
   are common   _____
5. Large muscles, very strong even if fat;
   one of the strongest of all types   _____
6. Teeth are large, irregular, white, or
   yellowish with age   _____
7. Wide fingers and toes (mostly males)   _____

8. Broad nose is common (males) _____
9. Male chest large; bust large _____
10. Face and chin large, wide, with a round-square shape _____
11. Straight dark eyebrows usually, some bushy; sunken eyes; many blue-eyed _____
12. Positive, frank, honest, plain-speaking _____
13. Great standing strength _____
14. Hair black, varied colors, wiry _____
15. Effective managers and supervisors _____
16. Unimpressed and don't back down if threatened _____
17. Dislike immorality and crudeness _____
18. Broad hips; expanded large abdomen is typical with age (especially males) _____
19. Highly developed sense of justice; may take revenge if wronged _____
20. Highly opinionated and skeptical _____
21. Very frank, outspoken, controlling _____
22. Respect and admire successful, power-ful, organized and efficient, people _____
23. Rational thinkers, few academics; usually learn wisdom from living life _____
24. Respect good deeds and friends _____
25. Very practical; high common sense _____
26. Highly modest _____
27. Good memory for things seen, heard, experienced; slow with book learning _____
28. Love right action and noble deeds _____
29. Hate inactivity; desire hard physical work and play _____

30. May be reckless without regard to
    own safety   _____
31. Are not naturally diplomatic   _____
32. Strong convictions; rarely change mind _____
33. Slow, deliberate, plain-speaking; read,
    act and express self honestly   _____
34. Practical, mechanical, skilled worker _____
35. Attracted to politics, managing, sports,
    supervising, music, or engineering _____
36. High common sense, decisiveness,
    modesty, independence   _____
37. Cannot tolerate dirt, smells, chemicals,
    sick people   _____
38. May not hold to orthodox religious
    beliefs; some may not believe in God,
    while others are fervent believers _____
39. Have very strong willpower   _____
40. Return good deed for good deed   _____
41. Are jocular; females more serious   _____
42. Tend to have cool verbal expression _____
43. History of joint pain or arthritis _____
44. Have courage of convictions;
    speak the truth bluntly   _____
45. Socially correct and obedient   _____
46. Addiction possible, but rare   _____
47. Deep feelings mostly under control _____
48. Self-actualizing, able to take action _____
49. Believe in being happy and optimistic _____
50. Head larger, bony, wide, square;
    forehead large, bony   _____
51. Impressed by honest talented people _____
52. Employees appreciate work-ethic   _____

53. Not moved by tears and emotions _____
54. Greatly respect self-controlled people _____
55. Mouth wide; teeth irregular, large _____
56. Expect obedience to their will _____
57. Do not tolerate fools well _____
58. Are logical and even-minded _____
59. Extremities strong, muscled; hands,
    feet (and toes) wide and strong _____
60. Highly practical and result-oriented _____
61. Strong durable joints when young;
    gout and arthritis with aging _____

Scoring

For question #1:
  A response: give 15 points = _____
  B response: give 7 points = _____
  C response: give 1 points = _____

For questions #2—61:
  A response: give 5 points = _____
  B response: give 3 points = _____
  C response: give 1 point   = _____

Total of the above points   = _____

Interpretation

151—285: PROBABLY Pallinomic type
80—150: POSSIBLY Pallinomic type
  <80:   NOT Pallinomic type

The Pallinomic Type

Rocine: "Pallinomic means 'potential for greatness'. You utilize more food <u>calcium, sodium, and carbon</u> than other types."

————

In the *palinomic* type, calcium and sodium make you a strong muscle type, while carbon (carbohydrates) predisposes you to becoming fat. You are typically medium-sized and muscular until about age 20, after which time you slowly gain weight, with many pot-bellied males.

If male, you occasionally stay medium-sized throughout life, but only with the right diet and exercise. Usually you don't watch your diet and inevitably eat yourself into a strong fatty body with an abdominal pot. You may end up looking like a fat type—but actually, you are a heavy muscle type! Excellent examples are John Wayne, Johnny Weismuller (Tarzan), President Lyndon Johnson, Ed McMann, Jane Russell and Rosemary Clooney (both of them were slender as young adults), and Attorney General Janet Reno. You are prudent, practical, conservative, modest, and self-actualizing: a person of action (when so motivated).

▶ *You may have raw courage and fearlessness; the males may enjoy hunting dangerous game—you enjoy taking risks! One man I knew would successfully hunt dangerous, wild pigs with just a knife and a dog.*

Physical Similarity to Other Types

The heavier *nitropheric* type (Dick Chenney, Marilyn Monroe) is medium or tall with less fat. As young adults you are commonly confused with them.

The *lipopheric* type (Rush Limbaugh, Ricki Lake) is fatter but may have a similar look. The *pallinomic* and *carboferic* types are usually pot-bellied).

The *oxypheric* type (Stephen Segal, Ella Fitzgerald) has a larger head and body, but is more outgoing, friendly, and intellectual.

The heavier *desmogenic* type (Marlon Brando, Madeleine Albright) is bony, and more intellectual and emotionally intense.

Average Height and Weight

Males:	5'10-6'8	170-300+ pounds
Females:	5'7-6'2	160-280+ pounds

You already know something about this type from their public persona and appearance, whether from seeing them yourself or from the celebrity examples. Blend such insights with the type descriptions and the types of your family and friends to discern their presence in your midst!

———

Pallinomic Type Description

The type description represents how you appear in everyday society. You may have a sub-type that alters parts of this description.

Think of the celebrity examples as you read the descriptions. You have a muscular body, but usually become portly with age. You display a large forehead and cheekbones, a square head, dark hair, wide mouth, muscular neck, large chest, pot belly, heavy limbs, and wide hands and feet—and a smart and practical brain.

Head — A large, bony, muscular, wide and square head with balanced features is usual; the forehead is larger than average.

Hair —Your hair is wiry, intense and strong; balding and graying is common with aging.

Eyes — Straight eyebrows are common, sometimes being quite bushy in males; the eyes are sunken with a prominent orbital bone surrounding them; many of you are blue-eyed.

Ears — The ears tend to be large, wide and irregularly shaped (particularly in the males).

Nose — A broad nose is common.

Face — Your face is large, wide and flat with large cheekbones; the chin is wide, with a round or square shape; the upper jaw is large.

Mouth and Lips — You have a wide mouth with normal lips. The voice is firm, confident, and authoritative.

Teeth — The teeth are large, irregular and white (or yellow from aging).

Neck — The neck is short, broad, strong, and fatty with age.

Skin — Your skin may have a peculiar tint (and odor). You commonly have freckles.

Muscles — You have strong and resilient muscles, making you one of the strongest types (along with *desmogenic, carbogenic, and Lipopheric* types).

▶ *I know several males who were exceedingly strong, all with large abdomens. In a garage, a car had fallen off its jack onto a mechanic, and a pallinomic man affected a rescue by lifting the car up!*

Chest — The male chest is large and strong, with minimal chest hair; the bust is large and often pendulous with age.

Back and Shoulders — A broad strong back and shoulders with great standing strength is common.

Hips and Abdomen — Broad and fatty hips are usual with an expanded abdomen in middle-age; the waist is large.

Arms and Legs —The extremities are strong, and well-padded with muscle and fat; males particularly have large fingers and toes.

Joints — Your joints are strong and durable when young, but due to your genetics and an excessively acid-ash diet (meats and carbo-hydrates) you tend to eventually suffer with arthritis and gout.

Fat — After being a slender teenager the female often starts becoming matronly in her twenties or thirties. The males are typically medium-sized and muscular until about age 20, after which time weight is slowly gained until you often manifest a pot-belly. Both sexes eat too much, and exercise too little. You easily may be mistaken for a *Fat* type—but you are a fat *Muscle* type!

———

Pallinomic Personality Traits

If you are this Muscle type many, but not all, of the following characteristics are present (you may have overcome or moderated the negatives, but should recognize that you once had several of them)

You may have any of the following traits:

- Aggressive in work and play
- High: self-confidence, image
- Self-confident, mostly humble
- Speak slowly, deliberately and plainly
- Have success potential, some are lazy
- Make excellent police, military officers
- Are passionate, tactful, guarded, controlled

- Are not hypocrites: very truthful and honest
- Usually consent when appealed to by reason
- Return good deeds for good (and bad for bad)
- Are positive, frank, plain-speaking, courageous
- Have very strong willpower, are result-oriented
- Deep feelings are under control (unless offended)
- Fearless of physical altercation (males particularly)
- Are polite and deferential, particularly to superiors
- Respect self-control, good deeds, and good friends
- Have a happy optimistic front (whether true or not)
- Have a confident ability to talk and interact with people
- Unimpressed by, do not back down if threatened by force
- Naturally active: inactivity is a pariah to you; enjoy hard work
- Good thinkers, rarely academic, learn and gain wisdom from life

- Have common sense, order, decisiveness, independence, modesty, and love of nature
- Strongly dislike evil, immorality, crudeness, betrayal, disobedience, rudeness, and laziness
- Are effective managers and supervisors: able to hire the right person for the right job
- Very strong love of home, mate, family; you strive for a true practical love and marriage
- Admire power, success, organization, efficiency, ethical people, powerful people, a strong work-ethic
- Good memory for things that can be seen, heard and experienced; poor memory for book learning
- Love right action, loyalty, noble deeds, mountains, hiking, antiquity, pets, music, dancing, philosophy, honor, metaphysics

▶ *Like the desmogenic and nitropheric males you may collect guns and use them wisely (many NRA members). The males want to feel safe and secure and to protect their turf.*

———

Potential Challenges

▶ *If you relate to any of these challenges, doing something to overcome them serves your evolution.*

You may have evolved from, or not experienced these general challenges, so don't dwell on them.

- Tend to be unforgiving if wronged
- May be lazy; are strongly opinionated
- High ideals, often disappointed in others
- May be indecisive at times and unable to act
- Often restless, stubborn, anxious to move on
- Antagonistic and grumpy if not getting own way
- Are not particularly social, sociable, or diplomatic
- Ready to help others with time, money and energy
- May be too frank, unfriendly, out-- spoken, skeptical
- Are never passive: erupt easily if crossed or disobeyed
- Cannot tolerate dirt, smells, chemicals, and sick people
- Tend to be overly-aggressive, defiant and plain speaking

- Have high sense of justice, may take revenge if wronged
- Some vulnerability to pot, alcohol or drug addiction; some resist it
- May leave a relationship suddenly (some dramatically so and are never heard from again); most are jealous
- Tend to be reckless in regard to personal safety (particularly males); females are also risk-takers

▶ *I know a few of you who enjoy hurting bad people and would love to be an avenger—if it was sociably or spiritually acceptable. You believe in an "eye for an eye" (like some nervimotives, pargenics, desmogenics, and medeics).*

───────

Pallinomic Stress Management

You have strong *mental* stress prevention givimg you a good ability not to internalize this stress into your stomach, adrenals, and immune system. This is because you have a very strong and balanced mental body. Your *emotional* stress prevention is variable, and the above challenges may need reprogramming help from the written releases described in Booklet #2.

───────

Love

Your love is true if love is returned; you seldom love more than once or twice, nor forgive any indiscretions by your mate. You are usually attracted to the *carboferic, carbogenic, eldic, marasmic, myogenic, and nitropheric* types. Sexual drive is strong.

———

Talents and Vocations

Abilities – *Military, police, sports, politics, teaching, supervisors, practical pursuits*

Your talent lies in try, try, try again until you succeed (just like Churchill, an *oxypheric*). You are skilled with hands and brain, and have a strong work ethic; you are managers of other people. You can do almost anything with your hands. I knew two karate instructors of your type: they were trim and fit—pure muscle with no obvious fat at all—a rare happening. To maintain a medium muscular figure you need a lifetime dedication to right eating and intensive exercise—but low self-discipline usually prevents this happening.

▶ *I have personally known you as auto-mechanics, policemen, physicians, teachers, detectives, karate experts, home-makers, dress-makers, biochemists; tennis, football, and baseball players...*

You thrive in politics because of your outspoken ideas, honesty, and ability to influence people. In the congress, senate, and presidency, President Johnson was very powerful with his networking and influence over politicians. The type information cannot predict what or who you will become, but you bring a creative excellence to whatever you do.

Inabilities - *Science, verbal eloquence, medicine*

Your mind doesn't turn easily to healing, compassion, or painstaking scientific applications. Although strong and fully capable, you don't do physical labor for long—you are leaders and supervisors!

Health Problems

If sick, you commonly experience health problems or diseases in any of the following organs and tissues:

Skeletal System and Joints — Your greatest weakness: arthritis and gout is commonly due to an erroneous diet.

Intestines — Are vulnerable to intestinal infections and diseases.

Kidneys and Liver — Are often inefficient from excessive protein or alcohol ingestion.

Vascular System — Diseased arteries or veins are common; the beef spokesmen on TV were often your type before their heart attacks. Exercise and sweats followed by deep massages are alkalinizing.

———

Pallinomic Acid/Alkaline Factor

[See the Appendix for details on this subject, along with the common symptoms found with people of different nervous system dominance.

For your health and healing, the genetics of your autonomic nervous system predispose you to needing a specific ratio of food acidity to alkalinity. You are born with an alkaline constitution, which means you need a predominantly **acid-ash** food intake (after metabolizing foods.) Your autonomic nervous system genetics are *parasympathetic* dominant, and theoretically, you need 70% acid-ash foods (proteins, carbohydrates) to 30% alkaline-ash, but you tend to eat excessively of acid-ash foods.

For your healing if in ill health, or after about age 40-45, you need to aim for this approximate ratio of food selections:
   50% Proteins, carbohydrates
   50% Fruits, salads, vegetables

▶ *Approximate your food ratios. On any particular day, it does not matter if one meal is mostly alkaline and another mostly acid—just try to balance it out for the day! If you make a mistake, try again tomorrow. It is a subjective call that you make, and what is done over time that makes the difference to your health.*

The Pallinomic Spiritual Factor

Skip this paragraph if uninterested in a philosophical perspective on your type!

If as souls, we choose the brain and body type to spend a lifetime in, it could be to learn certain spiritual lessons related to perfecting ourselves, and our humanity, in God's eyes. What lessons does the type bring you? If this type, only you can really decide what those lessons are. You know your weaknesses, faults, and behaviors towards others. You know things about yourself that Victor Rocine could never get from his research subjects when he first wrote about types. So search your mind for the answers.

Each discrete type has challenges of life lessons, spiritual goals, etc., and some of yours may be:

► *Rocine: "The soul chooses the body type."*

Faith — May be believers, or not! Some have a deep faith.

Unforgiving — When someone crosses you, you punish them—as difficult as it is, give yourself permission to forgive!

Too Frank and Outspoken — You express your feelings and thoughts easily, which may create relationship stress. You tend to be critical of others and of their behaviors. Get over it.

Arrogant, Aloof — You tend to feel superior to other people; consider if you really are in God's eyes?

Excessively Practical — You are overly practical, and for brain balance need right-brain activity like writing, creative arts or music daily.

Rest — Some of you are lazy, others always busy. Find the balance.

Ego Strength — You have a very strong ego. This coupled with your attitude and high self-acceptance and self-value, repels some people.

▶ *Those of you spiritually evolved have few, if any, of these negative qualities.*

———

A Pallinomic Story...

Hank, age 44, 6'3, strong, heavy, and pot-bellied, needed help with his fatigue, arthritis, and weight gain. Examination showed he was sixty pounds overweight. A review of his diet revealed excessive intake of calcium foods: Swiss and cheddar cheese, turnip greens, parsley, corn tortillas, dandelion greens, watercress, tofu, and dried figs. He had deficiencies in sodium foods (unsalted): fish, scallops, lobster, celery, Swiss chard, beets and greens, dulse, blackstrap molasses, rice bran, and cashews. Hank made the appropriate dietary changes along with the herbs indicated for his type, his weight steadily decreased, and his health improved.

———

Pallinomic Type
Mineral Foods

Apply this mineral data to the diet following these Muscle typedescriptions.

Excessive Foods:

- *Carbon (simple carbohydrates)*
- *Sodium (salted, junk)*
- *Calcium*
- *Uric Acid*

Deficient Foods:

- *Magnesium*
- *Potassium*
- *Sodium (unsalted, non-junk))*

These deficient nutrients are common deficiencies in your type, and predispose you to ill-health.

If ill, be sure to use these lists with your daily food intake. If not ill, eat from the foods lists 3-4 times weekly. All food lists are in descending order of concentration and value to you; choose servings of foods in the upper half of each list first!

One serving is ½ cup.

Pallinomic Excessive Foods -

Carbon is excessive so minimize its intake. It is excessive in all people who become fat or obese, and is in every cell of your body as the basis of life. You particularly need to minimize simple sugars (cookies, ice cream, candy, corn syrups, etc.).

Sodium from salted junk foods is excessive in your tissues. To preserve your health and weight control you should avoid junk foods and fulfill your sodium needs from the food list (without using the salt shaker; if you crave salt it indicates adrenal gland problems).

Calcium is excessive in your tissues. It is highly concentrated in your bones, joints, muscles, nerves, heart, teeth, and gums, and if you have an illness or disease in any of these tissues, calcium excess may be a significant problem. (This often requires a nutritionist aware of how environmental toxicity interferes with calcium metabolism.)

Uric Acid foods contribute to gout, to which you are vulnerable, so minimize them. See the following food list.

———

Deficient Foods -

In illness or disease, it is important to correct these mineral deficiencies.

Magnesium, deficient in your type, is particularly important for your heart and digestive function; deficiency links to diabetes, migraines, osteoporosis, heart disease, and high blood pressure.

Potassium is deficient in your type. It is the dominant element in your tissues and is concentrated in and vital to the health of your muscles, heart, brain, and all cells. If ill or diseased, potassium foods and supplements are probably a significant healing factor.

Sodium in unsalted food form is deficient (see above notes).

[See the Appendix for mineral descriptions.]

Note

Uric acid *(avoid these foods as they predispose you to gout):*

Roe, sweetbreads, heart, mussels, liver, kidney, pheasant, trout, veal, mutton, salmon, bacon, pork, ham, cod, crab, meat extracts, meat soups.

Minimize
Excessive Foods

Carbon (carbohydrates):
1-3 servings/week

Grains and breads, simple carbohydrates (white and brown sugars, high fructose corn syrup, honey, maple syrup, molasses, jellies, candy, ice cream, soda drinks).

Sodium (salted, junk): 0-1 servings/week

Salt, all fast foods, packaged foods, canned and frozen foods, soy sauce, all preserved meats (cured, smoked, canned and luncheon meats), sauces (barbecue, catsup, etc.), dill pickles, sauerkraut, bouillon cubes, peanut butter, potato chips, etc., salted nuts, crackers, canned or packaged soups, processed cheeses,.

Calcium: 2-3 servings/week only

Swiss and cheddar cheese, turnip greens, almonds, brewer's yeast, parsley, corn tortillas, dandelion greens, Brazil nuts, watercress, dried figs, yogurt, milk, sunflower seeds, whole wheat.

Eat
Deficient Foods

Magnesium, Potassium: *1-2 servings / day*

Bran, Swiss chard, oats, brown rice, lamb, turnips, molasses, kelp, cashews, filberts, peanuts, pecan, walnuts, rye, beet greens, soybean (cooked), sesame seeds, dried prunes, avocados.

Sodium (unsalted, non-junk):
1-2 servings / day

Kelp, blue and goat's cheese, strawberries, Swiss chard, beets and greens, lentils, oats, okra, poultry and gizzards, celery, salt water fish, lamb.

Note: Eat any other foods that you desire (not on these lists), but be sure to include the type foods in your daily choices.

Note -

The food recommendations are for the generic type. Additionally, you may need from a holistic healer or nutritionist something more specific for your individuality.

Pallinomic Nutritional Supplements

[Take all supplements with food.]

- **Multi-Vitamins** —
  2 capsules/day
- **Potassium** —
  99 mg/day
- **Minimize Calcium supplements**
  (Exception: menopause, on estrogen, or osteoporotic). You already have too much calcium in your tissues, absorbing it very easily and excessively, which contributes to your arthritis and hardening diseases.
- **Magnesium** —
  200 mg/day with food
- **Herbs** —
  *Brain detox – Gotu Kola or Ginkgo
  Organ detox – Milk Thistle or
                      Strawberry Leaf*
  Take one capsule, twice daily for one month; then three times weekly for maintenance.
- **Evening Primrose or Flaxseed Oil**
  1 soft-gel
  Note - Be sure to take these supplements if you have ill-health. If in good health, take them at least 3-4 times/week.

Important Pallinomic Health Concerns

Your nervous system genetics require the *Muscle* type Food Guide, which is fine while you are young. Strong carnivorous genetics cause you to eat excessively of red meats and dairy foods predisposing you to arthritis, gout, and disease. Eventually, you need a more *semi-vegetarian diet,* to restore and maintain your health.

You need the type mineral foods, complex carbohydrates, green salads and vegetables, limited red meat, and a diet high in unsalted sodium *foods,* with abundant water intake (especially after age 35), and **no** extra salt! Fish, poultry, and eggs are excellent for you several times weekly. You need to develop slower eating habits for better digestion.

Important Rocine Note

If unhealthy, Rocine recommended eating 1-3 servings of these two food categories <u>daily</u>:

<u>Citric</u> acid foods:

Grapefruit, citron, limes, oranges, pomegranate, raspberries

<u>Formic</u> acid foods:

Avocado, cucumbers, mangos, pears, persimmons, pineapples

[If in good health be sure to eat these foods regularly.]

PALLINOMIC FOOD GUIDE

Aim for -
50% Proteins, complex carbohydrates
50% Fruits, salads, vegetables
and
50% Raw foods
50% Cooked foods
Minimize dairy foods
Lose the salt shaker!
Follow the above advice from Rocine.

▶ *Rocine: "Like the calciferic type, you tend to overeat protein, milk, cheese, dairy, flesh and calcium foods until your organs and arteries are ossified and diseased with arteriosclerosis, arthritis, etc."*

———

Pallinomic Weight Loss

Broths of shell-fish, because of their high natural chloride content, are beneficial to your health and weight-loss. You have a good ability to lose and control your weight by following the Food Guide instructions. But, you do enjoy eating—use your willpower! Obviously, if you have a medical condition that contradicts this advice, do not change your diet!

- *Stop* eating carbon and sodium junk foods
- *Protein* drink daily, about 25-30 grams
- *Lose the salt shaker forever!*
- *Eat* your body type deficient mineral foods daily
- *Follow* your *Pallinomic Guide (as above)*
- *Exercise*: your body type requires moderately intense daily exercise
- *Simple sugars*: stop all white table sugar and high-fructose corn syrup and drinks containing these sugars
- *Calories:* As with any dietary approach, calories in, must be *less than* calories out! Most markets sell a calorie booklet; make notes of your daily intake, and in most instances keep it under about 1500 calories/day

———

Summary

Some muscle types appear to be *Fat* types, like the older male *desmogenic, myogenic, nitropheric, and you!* Some careful study allows you to discern the differences as these are heavy *Muscle* types—*not Fat types.*

———

Muscle Types
General Food Guide

(Carnivores)

Important Note

———

The Food Guide addresses the <u>Acid-Alkaline</u> aspect of your food intake, along with the <u>Type Mineral</u> factor presented throughout this book. It does <u>not</u> necessarily address calories or other dietary factors that may be pertinent to your personal health needs whether medical or appropriate for some other dietary need. So use your common sense and just include the factors described here with whatever healthy dietary choices you usually make.

For other nutrient information, consult with nutritional books or with holistic nutritional doctors. I particularly recommend the advice of Andrew Weil, M.D.

———

General Food Guide

*This is a **general** Food Guide, upon which you superimpose the nutritional information from your type chapter. As a Muscle body type, your genetics require flesh foods. (Note that a Thin sub-type would move you towards being vegetarian.)*

———

Meat/Flesh Intake

Most muscle types should limit red meat to once or less weekly, while eggs, lamb, fish, or poultry are excellent in moderation. If ill or diseased, be sure to eat daily, one or two servings from each *deficient minerals* list. If not ill, eat them at least three times weekly for health maintenance. If this diet is similar to your present diet, but healing is sluggish, then:

- Decrease your carbohydrate and protein intake by about one-third
- Increase your fruit, salad, and vegetable intake by about one-third
- Consult with a holistic doctor, preferably one versed in nutritional and emotional evaluation

———

Over-Acid or Over-Alkaline?

Just as a log of wood burned in your fireplace leaves a mineral-ash, food ash refers to the minerals remaining after metabolizing foods in your tissues:

- Fruits and vegetables ***alkalinize*** tissues
- Proteins and carbohydrates ***acidify*** tissues

Usually You Are Over-Acid Due To:

- Excessive intake: dairy foods
- Excessive intake: proteins, carbohydrates
- Deficient intake: fruits, vegetables
- Accumulated metabolic waste-acids (from years of eating excessive meats and carbohydrates, and lack of exercise)
- Estimate the ratio of foods eaten. Generally, eat the following *approximate* ratio of foods for your health:

50% **Alkaline-ash** foods *(fruits, salads, vegetables)*

50% **Acid-ash** foods *(complex carbo-hydrates like starches, grains, cereals, breads, flour products; and proteins)*

Approximate your food ratios. On any particular day, it does not matter if one meal is mostly alkaline, and another mostly acid—just try to balance it out for the day! If you get it wrong, try again tomorrow. It is a subjective call that you make, and it is what you do over weeks, months, or years that make the difference—not on any one or two days or weeks.

———

Note - If Vegetarian

As a general indication, if you follow a vegetarian diet substitute vegetable sources of protein for the any flesh in the food guide. Note that contrary to most alkaline-ash vegetarian diets you need something different:

*You need an **acid-ash** vegetarian diet high in complex carbohydrates and vegetable proteins.*

Because of your high need for protein, you usually require a daily vegetable powdered protein supplement in juice (about 25-30 grams).

———

Important

- Minimize white sugar and alcohol intake.
- If desired, interchange lunches for dinners.

- Never eat foods you are allergic to, no matter what I recommend; if allergic, or suspect a food allergy, eliminate it and substitute from your type mineral lists.

- Eat the right foods 80-90% of the time and the Food Guide will work for you; unlike some types you do not have to live out of a health food store (although such foods are healthier for you).

▶ *Omit eating the excessive minerals in your type chapter, and be sure to eat one or two servings from the deficient list daily.*

Finally, in addition to your body type needs, other holistic healing matters also need your attention. I strongly suggest that you refer to my web site and earlier books for that information: *DrStenbeck.net*

————

Acid/Alkaline Genetics Chart

The following chart reflects each Muscle Type needs for acid or alkaline-ash foods. These ratios change if you are unhealthy or over age 45-50. Refer back to your body type and review the *Acid/alkaline* instructions.

————

Acid/Alkaline Genetics, Dietary-Ash, and Raw Food Needs

This chart shows the Rocine types, their acid or alkaline food needs, and the percentage of raw foods needed for your health and healing.

- Apply your Type Minerals to the Food Guide

Type Genetics	Acid/Alkaline Needed	% Food-Ash Needed	% Raw Food
Calciferic	Alkaline	70% acid	30
Carbogenic	Alkaline	50-50	50
Desmogenic	Alkaline	70% acid	50
Eldic	Intermediate	50-50	50
Medeic	Intermediate	50-50	50
Myogenic	Intermediate	50-50	50
Nervimotive	Alkaline	70% acid	50
Nitropheric	Acid	70% alkaline	70
Pallinomic	Alkaline	50-50	30

The above percentages vary depending on aging and the health of individual types.

General Food Guide
Breakfast

Use the nutritional information from your Type Chapter everyday in this Guide.

EGGS* (1-2) with lettuce, tomato, or salad, whole grain toast; (add bacon or sausage 1-3 times weekly if desired) — 2-4 times/week; or

FRUIT fresh salad, and protein (yogurt, milk, cheeses, seeds, nuts) —1-3 times/week; or

CEREALS, with fruit, seeds, nuts —2-5 times/week; or

OTHER choices — 0-1 times weekly

Daily liquids:
Pure water, citrus, vegetable juices, soups, other —as desired
Coffee, teas —0-2 cups

Lunch

*SALADS, mixed green, protein
(poultry, fish, egg, cheese, seeds or nuts, etc.),
whole grain breads
[Dressing: olive oil/ vinegar; low-fat, low-cal
dressings]
— 2-4 times/week; or*

*SANDWICH, whole grains with a
protein (cheese, tuna, ham, etc.); and salad
and/ or vegetables
— 1-4 times/week; or*

*POULTRY, FISH, 3-6 oz., with a
mixed green salad and/ or vegetables
—1-3 times/week; or*

*OTHER choices (with salad or vegetables)
—1-2 times/week*

*[Other oils are permitted, but less ideal:
soybean oil is a common allergen; minimize
commercial dressings. Be sure to include two
or more selections from your type food lists in
your daily food intake. For in-between meal
snacks, eat fruit or vegetables with
seeds/ nuts.]*

Dinner

POULTRY, FISH (4-6 oz.), with salad and/or vegetables
—2-4 times/week; or

PASTA with protein (chicken, etc.) with salad and/or vegetables
— 2-4 times/week; or

VEGETARIAN meal with salad and/or vegetables
—1-3 times/week; or

LEAN BEEF (4-6 oz.) with salad and/or vegetables
— 0-1 times/week

OTHER choices with salad and/or vegetables
— 0-1 times/week

Desserts:
Fruits, fresh —as desired
Low-sugar, healthy desserts
— 0-3 times/wk

Food Guide Notes

Steamed Vegetables —

Minerals are lost in the boiling of vegetables; steaming or wok cooking is best.

Food Combinations —

If you have a weak digestive system then eating proteins at the same meal with starches often results in indigestion, gas, or constipation.

Periodic Detox —

You tend to over-indulge in acid-ash foods (proteins and carbohydrates), and often need occasional elimination diets for tissue waste-acid removal. Have a holistic doctor or nutritionist supervise such detox (where you have an alkaline-ash diet along with protein supplementation).

Minimize —

- Fatty foods
- Commercial salad dressings
- Beef, red meats, processed meats
- Coffee, white sugar, corn syrup, alcohol

Vegetarian Proteins —

You require a carnivorous diet. The exception is the *nitropheric* type who functions best with a *vegetarian* diet; the other muscle types are born to be carnivores. It is very difficult for the other muscle types to be pure vegetarians because of their strong intuitive cravings for fish, poultry, meat, or eggs. If you are vegetarian, then because of your high needs for amino acids and acid-ash foods, you should take a protein supplement of 30-40 grams/day (powdered protein in juice).

Healthy Weight —

Several of you gain weight as the ravages of age, lack of exercise and dietary excesses take their toll. By eating according to your body type, you should naturally lose excess weight. Each type also has a few individual factors that only apply to them!

You have a good ability to lose weight by following the Food Guide instructions. The most common problem I find with your weight-control is liver and kidney irritation due to food allergies, which results in extra pounds. The key is to eat non-allergic foods.

If drinking more than 3-4 cups daily of coffee or tea, you may have a hypoglycemic problem (low blood sugar), which contributes to making fat, ill-health, and delayed healing. (Refer to the earlier books for help with this healing.)

In some *Fat* types, like the lean or medium-sized young adult *isogenic and pargenic*, you may be inclined to call them *Muscle* types: study them carefully to discern the differences.

* * *

Appendix

Brief Extracts from
<u>The 22 Unique Body Types</u>

Appendix A

Types
(Brief extract)

Type comes from 'typus' meaning an image or impression, the study of types being called typology.

▶ *Rocine: "A combination of mental and structural features is consistently found in people of the same type."*

Rocine wrote that all types are a mixture of positive and negative qualities. He based his work on the biochemical individuality of our *mineral* absorption and utilization. Of course, all minerals are absorbed, but he postulated that different types of people *selectively* absorb certain minerals, to a greater or lesser extent, requiring specific mineral foods for their enhanced health and healing.

▶ *The type information cannot predict what or who you will become, or how successful or not, but your type is capable of bringing a creative excellence to whatever you do in life. If your type has negative qualities that you disagree with, remember that they are only tendencies and may or may not manifest in you.*

This book enlarges on Rocine's premise (early 1900's), integrated with the later research of Herbert Sheldon, M.D., Ph.D., at Harvard University (1930's), along with my fifty years of observations and experience with this subject.

Comparing your shared physical (and sometimes psychological) descriptions with the Celebrity Lists further assists the identification of your type. It is not that you will look exactly like, or be a twin to, any particular celebrity. Look closely at a celebrity's features: face, profile, height, weight, head, etc. If you know something about their talents, beliefs, success and failure spheres, health and weight challenges, attitudes and behaviors, etc., then you get clues as to what your type may be.

———

Understanding Types and Sub-Types

Each of us has a clearly discernible dominant type. Visualize the celebrity examples from movies, politics, sports, the arts and public life, and try to identify with their physical features. Look for similar features, remembering that you will not recognize all attributes in yourself. You are not looking for your twin!

The sub-type issue is the main reason people of the same major type can look so different. Remember that a type description does not characterize you exactly, but depicts your individual variant of a type.

▶ *The type questionnaire pinpoints the major features of that type: if the celebrity examples are unhelpful, you may be an unusual variant (in which case ignore the celebrity issue and give yourself 7 points on Question 1).*

———

Minerals

Minerals are essential life nutrients that accelerate enzyme and chemical reactions and provide a basis for your body typing. Although found in all tissues, different minerals tend to be concentrated in certain organs, their presence or absence contributing to the healing of such tissues; e.g., zinc accelerates prostate healing; calcium and manganese promote bone, joint and connective tissue healing.

Specific foods nurture each type, some people needing meats for their health others needing a vegetarian diet. A high potassium diet nurtures one person, while another needs high sulfur, calcium, zinc, or another mineral.

Mineral Digestion and Absorption

Compared to vitamins, minerals are *difficult* to digest, absorb, and utilize. In people with strong digestive systems, this aspect may not be important. The following factors should be in place for optimal mineral metabolism:

1. Stomach Hydrochloric Acid Production
2. Parathyroid Hormone Balance
3. Organ Toxic Metal and Chemical Removal
   [See details in The 22 Unique Body Types.]

―――――

Total Body Healing

Note that from a holistic healing perspective, in addition to minerals and type information, the following healing factors are necessary:

> *Nutrient Balance*
> *Mental Balance*
> *Emotional Balance*
> *Spiritual Balance*
> *Detoxifying Integrity*

The above factors are all important to your total healing especially if you are interested in self-healing (see my earlier books).

―――――

Appendix B

Researchers
(Brief extract)

The predominant workers in this area of human individuality from around 1880's to the 1960's are Herbert Sheldon, M.D., Ph.D., Roger Williams, Ph.D., and Victor Rocine, D.Sc.

Much information on Sheldon's research exists on-line and in medical psychology libraries; for interested readers there are other lines of research published in the last century. This present book is primarily about Rocine's body types.

Herbert Sheldon M.D., Ph.D.

In contrast to Rocine, Sheldon at Harvard University in the 1930's was trained in the scientific method and did painstaking research and publishing on human individuality. In comparing his findings with Rocine's work, a direct putative correlation is visible.

Roger J. Williams, Ph.D.

Another significant researcher in human individuality is the renowned scientist and biochemist, Roger J. Williams. He demonstrated that different people have varying levels of nutrients, enzymes, and other metabolic chemicals in their bloodstreams.

▶ *Williams's research firmly expands on the premise of individual nutritional needs in human beings. If interested in his research, I highly recommend his book Biochemial Individuality.*

Victor Rocine, D.Sc.

Note that when a negative feature is indicated, say neurotic tendencies, all members of the type are <u>not</u> that way; it is a type tendency reported by Rocine.

Rocine studied type-related diseases finding links between mineral and dietary factors with individual types and their diseases. In each body type, one or more dominant minerals are preferentially absorbed and utilized over other minerals.

He recognized discrete body types from their physical appearance finding genetically based mineral dominance to be the determining feature. He also correlated their physical features with psychological characteristics.

———

Appendix C

Genetics, Types, and Diet
(Brief extract)

This section deals with how nervous system genetics helps determine your eating choices for health: you are either born to be a predominant meat eater, a partial or complete vegetarian, or something between the two. The genetic factor determining this dietary aspect is the *sympathetic and parasympathetic* components of your central nervous system. This represents a basic factor in eating for health.

This chapter helps you understand your dietary inheritance, although instinctively, you may already have arrived there!

- If born **sympathetic** dominant you are *genetically acid*, desiring a predominantly *vegetarian* diet for your health (about 70% fruit, salad, vegetables to 30% proteins and carbohydrates).

- If born **parasympathetic** dominant you are *genetically alkaline*, desiring a predominantly *carnivorous* diet for your health (about 70% proteins, carbohydrates to 30% fruits, salads, vegetables). Few of you ever choose to become vegetarian because of the difficulty in satisfying your protein needs without meats.

- If born ***intermediate*** dominant you may eat food groups with little concern for the acid/alkaline factor. However, after age 40, you need a semi-vegetarian diet for healthy eating.

———

Chart of Relative Nervous System Dominance

In the following Chart, if you relate to many of the symptoms on one side you probably have that nervous system dominance; relating to both sides indicates *Intermediate* dominance.

If Vegetarian (Over-acid) --
> *Eat 70% fruits, salads, vegetables*
> *And 30% proteins, carbohydrates*

If Carnivore (Over-alkaline) --
> *Eat 70% proteins, carbohydrates*
> *And 30% fruits, salads, vegetables*

If Intermediate --
> *Eat 50:50 of acid and alkaline-ash foods*

Make an *approximate* estimate of your daily acid and alkaline food intake (such ratios varying from type to type).

———

Symptoms of Relative Genetic Dominance

Vegetarians (Over-acid)	Carnivores (Over-alkaline)
Sympathetic Dominance	Parasympathetic Dominance
little or no flesh desire	desire flesh
easily constipated	rarely constipated
slow digestion	fast digestion
easily dehydrated	not dehydrated
strong thirst	low thirst
pale face	flushed face
high pulse after food	slow pulse after food
easy gag reflex	slow gag reflex
cool dry skin	moist warm skin
nervous stomach	calm stomach
little eyelid blinking	much blinking
nervous tendency	mostly calm
slower healing	faster healing
low oxygen-uptake	good oxygen-uptake
easily breathless	seldom breathless
insomnia common	sleep easier
few muscle cramps	some night cramps
calcium deposits rare	get calcium deposits

Appendix D

Help Identifying your Body Type with Dr. Stenbeck

If you desire help in identifying your body type, follow these instructions, and answer the questionnaire. For further information and fees, send me an email from page one of the website:

DrStenbeck.net

First name: _____

Country of birth: _____

Upload photos and send to the above website:

- ■ Head and shoulders: front and side views

- ■ Full body: front and side views

- ■ Also 1-2 teenage views

- ■ If possible, casual photos of mother, father, siblings

MY TYPE CLASS MAY BE - _____

    (Thin, Muscle, or Fat)

AGE   -   _____

HEIGHT   -   _____ feet/inches

MY WEIGHT -   _____ pounds

    Heaviest at age: _____

- Lightest as adult: _____

- Estimate age 15: _____

VISION - Excellent Average   Poor:

HAIR - Natural color: _____

    - Thin/thick?   _____

    - balding?   _____

SKIN - Quality: _____

    - History of acne, boils, other:

_____

_____

TEETH   - Strong   Weak Dentures

    - Cavity history: Many   Moderate   Few

MUSCLES - Strong   Average   Weak

    Sports played _____

JOINTS   - Strong   Average   Weak

HEALTH - Childhood diseases?

_____

_____

- Adult diseases?

_____

AVERAGE DIET

- Beef   _____ (times/week)

 - Poultry   _____ (times/week)

 - Fish   _____ (times/week)

 - Eggs   _____ (times/week)

 - Water   _____ (glasses/day):

 - Vegetarian? Vegan?   _____

 - Other?   _____

 - Did your childhood diet differ? _____

The above will help me know who you are! I will send you a follow-up questionnaire for further help in identifying your body type.

Appendix E

On-line Health Consultation with Dr. Stenbeck

For further information, or to comment on this book, or to receive a response on any health issue from a holistic viewpoint, send an email inquiry from page one of my website:

DrStenbeck.net

Following that, I will suggest further healing needs, which we may pursue with an on-line consult.

————

Appendix F

Notes

See my book *The 22 Unique Body Types,* available at the usual online source, for further information and details on all of the 22 Types. The Appendix in that book has further information about:

Mineral Functions and Food Sources

Further Reading

———